THE HEALTH BEYOND THE SCALE PLANNER

90 DAYS OF JOURNAL PROMPTS AND COACHING EXERCISES FOR IMPROVING YOUR HEALTH WITHOUT DIETING

Karen Lynne Oliver, BA, MA
Founder of *Beyond the Bathroom Scale*®

Copyright © 2020 by Karen Lynne Oliver

All rights reserved. No part of this publication may be reproduced, distributed, or transmitted in any form or by any means, including photocopying, recording, or other electronic or mechanical methods, without the prior written permission of the author, except in the case of brief quotations embodied in critical reviews and certain other non-commercial uses, permitted by copyright law.

For permission requests, please email the author via the address below:

karenoliver@beyondthebathroomscale.co.uk

"*Beyond the Bathroom Scale*" is a Registered UK Trademark and the intellectual property of Karen Lynne Oliver, trading as *Beyond the Bathroom Scale®*, part of Lynne Media ('our', 'we', 'us').

We take the protection of our intellectual property very seriously. If we discover that you have breached the terms of the licence (as linked to in the footer above), we may bring legal proceedings against you and seek monetary damages and/or an injunction to stop you using our materials. You could also be ordered to pay our legal costs.

ISBN: 9798652580315
Imprint: Independently published for Lynne Media
Cover Image: Canva

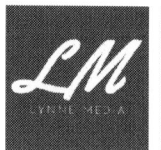
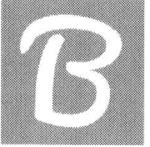

LEGAL DISCLAIMER

By continuing to use this planner you acknowledge and agree to the full disclaimer.

This planner is not appropriate for people with active eating disorders; if you are suffering from an eating disorder or have suffered from one in the past please seek professional advice from your GP instead.

Although this planner is intended to help heal your body image, it may be triggering for anyone who has an underlying eating disorder or illness such as body dysmorphia.

For Educational and Informational Purposes Only

The information provided in or through this Website is for educational and informational purposes only and solely as a self-help tool for your own use.

Not a Substitute for Professional Advice

I am not a registered therapist, dietitian, personal trainer, or any other kind of health professional and do not hold myself out to be. The information contained in this Website is not intended to be a substitute for health or wellbeing advice that can be provided by your own GP or health and wellbeing practitioner. The advice found on this Website should be treated as a suggestion, based on my own personal experience of what works for me, rather than from medical training. This programme is not a substitute for seeking professional help with eating disorders or other mental health issues.

Although care has been taken in preparing the information provided to you, I cannot be held responsible for any errors or omissions, and I accept no liability whatsoever for any loss or damage you may incur. Always seek health care advice from a registered professional, relating to your specific circumstances as needed for all questions and concerns you now have, or may have in the future. You agree that the information in this planner and on the website is not professional health care advice.

For everyone who wants to improve their physical health, without starting a war on food and their bodies.

The Health Beyond the Scale Planner

ABOUT THE AUTHOR

Karen Lynne Oliver, BA, MA, is the founder of *Beyond the Bathroom Scale®*, a hub of self-help resources to aid with recovery from disordered eating and body image.

Beyond the Bathroom Scale® was awarded 'Most Innovative Digital Health Business, UK' in 2020 by Acquisition International.

A former Social Worker, Karen holds a bachelor's degree in Sociology, specialising in health and society and a master's degree in Social Work. She has trained in counselling skills and psychotherapy-based approaches including Cognitive Behavioural Therapy (CBT), Dialectical Behavioural Therapy (DBT) and Motivational Interviewing (MI).

Karen has previously written for *HuffPost UK* and has been featured in *The Metro, Calm Moment, The Cambridge Independent* and *Cosmopolitan Magazine*.

FREE RESOURCES

Over on *Beyond the Bathroom Scale*® you can sign up to a **free six-day course** which includes 6 video lessons, a PDF workbook, and a guide to recommended resources.

The free six-day course covers:

1. What we mean by diet culture, how to recognise it, why it's harmful to your health and how to rebel against it.

2. Why self-compassion and body acceptance is essential for health.

3. How to listen to what your body is trying to tell you it needs most.

4. The causes behind emotional eating and the strategies for tackling it.

5. What is meant by Intuitive Eating and how it can help you gain freedom from dieting and improve your relationship with food and your body.

6. What the Health at Every Size® (HAES) movement is all about and the body of research which supports taking an anti-diet approach to improving physical health.

You can sign up for free and get started straight away using this link:

https://www.beyondthebathroomscale.co.uk/health-mindset-starter-kit

USEFUL LINKS:

- **[FREE] The Health Mindset Starter Kit:**
  https://www.beyondthebathroomscale.co.uk/health-mindset-starter-kit

- **[FREE] BTBS Community Support Facebook Group:**
  https://www.facebook.com/groups/btbsblog/

- **The Health Mindset Programme™:**
  https://www.beyondthebathroomscale.co.uk/thehealthmindsetprogramme/

- **Facebook Page:**
  https://www.facebook.com/BeyondTheBathroomScale/

- **Instagram:**
  https://www.instagram.com/beyondthebathroomscale

HOW TO USE THIS PLANNER

In the *Health Beyond the Scale Planner*, we will be taking steps to improve our physical health, without focusing on weight. The truth is, we can only truly focus on our health (both physical and psychological), when we have totally removed ourselves from diet culture and the dieting mindset.

Throughout this planner I want you to keep in mind that while our health is important, it is not a measure of our self-worth. It does not define us as people, as we are not 'bad' people when we become ill or if we have health issues.

This planner is split into three parts:

- **Part 1 - Joyful Movement**, where we will look at how to add pleasurable forms of movement into our lives, and work through the barriers and issues we may have around exercise.

- **Part 2 - Gentle Nutrition**, where we will look at the physical effect food has on us, some general nutritional guidelines (not rules!), and why calories and portion sizes are irrelevant. We will also discuss what we mean by the term 'play-food' and the value of 'play-food'.

- **Part 3 - Alternative Ways to Assess Health,** where we will look at biomarkers such as blood pressure, blood glucose and blood cholesterol. All of these are far more useful in diagnosing, managing, and preventing common lifestyle illness, than simply stepping on a bathroom scale. We'll also look at alternative ways to improve overall health.

If you'd like to know more about the anti-diet approach, intuitive eating and cognitive behavioural therapy, please visit my website at **https://www.beyondthebathroomscale.co.uk** and sign up for the **FREE 6-day course** on making peace with food and body.

Each section of this planner starts with coaching exercises and has 30 days of daily planner pages tailored to the goals of each of the three section. The daily planner pages also have sections for recording your mood and gratitude journaling.

Logging your mood can be useful for highlighting the link between your body image and your mood. For example, when we're happy about something, we may be less focused on our bodies. Likewise, our body image can impact our mood, so we may feel sad, anxious, or withdrawn on days where we feel low about our bodies.

A daily gratitude practice can help interrupt the seemingly never-ending stream of anxious thinking we can find ourselves trapped in when our stress levels are too high (known as ruminating). The simple act of taking one minute each day to write down three things you are grateful for (even small things like the weather, or someone letting you out of a busy junction) can really improve your mood by helping to put negative events into perspective and reminding you that life does have beauty in it, even in depths of the toughest of times.

WHAT DOES 'HEALTH BEYOND THE SCALE' MEAN?

Readers of my blog, **Beyond the Bathroom Scale®** and students on my courses and programmes, will already be aware of my disdain for the diet industry, including the media that supports and advertises on its behalf.

In particular, I take issue with the way the diet industry, media and mass marketing sets out to make women feel self-conscious, ugly and 'fat', in order to sell them apparent 'fixes' that they don't need (and don't work anyway). The bottom line is that someone profits big time from making women feel insecure about themselves. Sometimes this is even done in the name of promoting health, which riles me up further.

Health is *not* about appearance and it cannot be measured using a bathroom scale. There is an increasing amount of medical research to stand by this claim too.

In magazines and on social media, "fitness inspiration" is used as an incognito way of saying "slim, toned, young, white, feminine, aesthetically pleasing to the male gaze". It is diet culture sneaking under the radar, and while it's not overtly telling you to lose weight, it's still telling you that you need to drastically alter your appearance in order to be healthy or physically 'fit'.

As you can imagine, this ideal image alienates a lot of women who do not fall into these categories, often putting them off from taking an interest in fitness. In this planner, we will define exactly what 'health' really means.

Having come from academic background in Sociology and Psychology, I am all too aware of how media messages intertwine with our cultural values and our internal processes. Our relationship with food becomes fraught with anxiety over calories, macros, points, Syns, and different chemicals. We restrict food groups and amounts, and everything we do, drink, and eat is tracked, analysed, and picked apart.

Our movement is thought of as a workout, with the primary purpose or burning calories, "blasting fat", and "shredding our bodies", rather than being viewed as joyful activity.

All of this is done in the pursuit of changing our bodies, with the hope that in doing so, we will lead to a better life.

These actions may not even change your weight or overall health for the long term, let alone your life.

There's a very worrying tendency in our society to start a diet or follow an eating plan, lose some weight, binge/ have a cheat day/ or 'come off plan'/ and gain weight as a consequence, and then declare the start of another diet. It is seen as normal in fact, and is often joked about with colleagues at work, friends on a night out and even as an entire nation after Christmas. This is not only harmful to our physical health but is a precursor for disordered eating and eating disorders.

When you look at some of the habits diet culture promotes, it's easy to see how dieting can be a precursor to developing full blown eating disorders.

The diet-binge-diet cycle is painfully similar to the patterns of Binge Eating Disorder. So much so, that dieting, and restriction has been shown to drastically increase the chance of developing Binge Eating Disorder, among other types of eating disorders.

- Over-exercising may be used a way of 'purging' calories, as with bulimia nervosa, where laxatives or self-induced vomiting may be used. Restricting calories, coupled with an obsession with weight loss, underpins the foundation of anorexia nervosa.

- A preoccupation with nutrition, whereby becoming obsessed with the ingredients and nutritional values of everything you eat, can slide into Orthorexia or food phobias.
- And a disordered relationship with food and exercise, combined with a lack of self-care and regard for our emotional health, is also congruent with common issues like emotional eating, whereby we eat to numb our emotions or cheer ourselves up.

All of these have far more serious implications for our health (both physical and mental), than being overweight does.

This planner is designed to help you improve your physical health without resorting to dieting or having any focus on weight. In other words: improve your health beyond the bathroom scale.

INITIAL EXERCISES

'Health' is so much more than the number on the scale

HEALTH BEYOND THE SCALE SELF-ASSESSMENT

To begin, let's run through a quick exercise to get some idea of how well you're looking after your overall health and wellbeing. Read through the statements below and tick the ones you agree with or feel apply to you most of the time.

I attend dentist, optician and doctors' appointments and check-ups whenever required.	
I am aware of my blood pressure, blood glucose, and cholesterol readings, or I get these regularly checked/monitored.	
I do not intentionally diet or weigh myself.	
Most of the time I do not allow myself to become either too hungry or too full throughout the day.	
I do not restrict particular foods or food groups (except for allergy or religious reasons).	
I take part in exercise on a regular basis which I find enjoyable.	

I make sure I get plenty of sleep at night.	
I drink plenty of water throughout the day to stay hydrated	
I have in place a network of family and friends who support me.	
I have in place a self-care routine and different hobbies which I use to manage my mental health and stress levels.	

Tally up the number of ticks and make a note of your score below. We'll repeat this self-assessment again at the end of the planner to see how far you've progressed. The higher the score, the more you're doing to care for your health.

Today's date	
My score	

SECTION 1: JOYFUL MOVEMENT

Exercise to celebrate what your body can do, not to punish it for how it looks or for what you ate.

WHAT IS JOYFUL MOVEMENT?

In this part of the planner, we're going to discuss what we mean by joyful movement and why pleasure and joy is an important part of physical activity.

'Joyful movement' refers to any type of exercise or physical activity that makes us feel happy, joyful, or calm. It makes us feel good and boosts our mood. This might be a workout, some form of play or just general activity in the day.

Why is it important to find some type of movement that makes us feel joyful? According to hedonic motivation theory, we are more likely repeat something that brings us joy, and of course, regular exercise has many health benefits.

We're also less likely to view physical activity as a chore or a way of punishing our bodies, which is crucial when we're recovering from the dieting mindset and disordered eating.

Reference: Kaczmarek, Lukasz (2017) 'Hedonic Motivation', Encyclopaedia of Personality and Individual Differences, Publisher: Springer, Editors: V. Zeigler-Hill, T.K. Shackelford
https://www.researchgate.net/publication/315645306_Hedonic_Motivation

HEALTH BENEFITS OF JOYFUL MOVEMENT

Regular exercise has many benefits and can make huge difference to your overall health. It's important to point out that when people talk about the 'benefits of weight loss', many (if not all) of these benefits can be achieved through joyful exercise and gentle nutrition, so there's no need to suddenly start focusing on weight in order to improve our health.

Let's look at some of the many physical and psychological benefits of movement:

- **Reduction in health risks** - decreased risk of diabetes type 2, hypertension, stroke, bone fractures, osteoporosis, heart disease and many types of cancer (colon, endometrial, lung).
- **Short term improvements** (you'll benefit from these day to day and it doesn't take long at all to see improvements in these areas)- strength, mobility, range of movement, balance, cardio vascular improvements and stamina, sleep quality, and appetite regulation, as exercise helps to balance the hormonal disruption causes by food restriction.
- **Long term improvements** (these take a while to accumulate) - improved bone density, lower resting heart rate and blood pressure, lower cholesterol, improved digestion, and improved circulation.
- **Psychological and mental health** - boosts mood, clears mind, improves focus, boosts self-esteem, reduces symptoms of anxiety and depression, improves memory.

Take a few moments to jot down what you'd like to gain from exercise and how you would like it to feel afterwards. For example, do you want it to make you feel calmer, stronger, or more energized. This task will help you set your intentions for what you would like to achieve later in the section.

What do I want to get from exercise?

How do I want to feel after exercising?

BARRIERS TO EXERCISE

Even when we're aware of how good exercise is for us, many of us still struggle to add physical activity into our lives. Remember: we are specifically focusing on pleasurable forms of exercise – not self-punishing 6am bootcamp workouts! None the less, there can still be many barriers to physical activity, and we'll address these in this section.

COMMON BARRIERS TO EXERCISE

Let's discuss the most common barriers to exercise. Some people find it physically uncomfortable, this may be down to incorrect posture, pre-exciting health conditions or injuries, or (like teenage me!) even something as simple has a poorly fitted sports bra.

They may also just don't enjoy it, or rather, they haven't yet discovered a type of movement they do enjoy and have a very narrow idea of what counts as exercise.

They may dislike the environment it's carried out in, a gym or outside, for example. I know that for me personally; I can't stand the idea of exercising in all weathers. I hate the rain and wind (which we get a lot of in the UK!) so I prefer indoor workouts.

Other people dislike the idea of exercising in front of others at a gym studio or in a class and would prefer to exercise alone, either outdoors or at home. I started out exercising at home using dance video games for the Wii and Xbox Kinect, which gradually built my confidence up to the point of becoming a member of a gym and local pool.

They may also have a negative association of exercise because of a past experience. This too was a major concern for me, as I associated exercising with high school PE lessons, which I hated and would often bunk off because they embarrassed me so much.

Finally, a very important one to consider, differences in abilities, disabilities, and injuries can be a huge barrier for many people. Some types of exercise may not be appropriate for health reasons or require adaptation. If this is the case, I highly recommend seeking advice from your health professional (whether your GP or physiotherapist) and a personal trainer or qualified instructor.

On the next page, there is an exercise to help you identify your own barriers to exercise. Reading through each area, tick yes for barriers that apply to you. Rate each of the barriers you ticked, giving them a score between 1 and 5, with 1 being a minor concern, 5 being a major concern.

AREA OF CONCERN	YES	SCORE (1-5)
Mindset - Viewing it as punishment/ a way to lose weight / change your body		
Negative associations – Memories of school PE lessons/gym classes		
Environment – outside weather conditions, gym, exercising in public, group exercise or lone		
Time - fitting it around your schedule - how much time you have/ how you would fit into your routine		
Equipment and clothing – whether any special equipment is required (weights, yoga mat, running trainers)		
Budget – Cost of gym membership, PTs, group class fees, online subscriptions		
Physical ability - Disabilities, injuries, knowledge or how to safely perform exercise		

Next, we're going to tackle your barriers. Take any barriers you've rated 5 or 4 and spend some time thinking how you could overcome them. Note down your thoughts in your workbook.

Here are some examples to help you...

- **Time** - fitting movement into your general routine, gym opening hours, PTs that come to your house, online workout programmes, YouTube videos for 5-15-minute sessions, apps for 7 min cardio sessions.

- **Budget** – free exercise like running, walking, and hiking, dancing in your room, yoga vids on YouTube, cheap group class DVDs, online subscription cheaper than gym, car boot sales and eBay for equipment

- **Negative associations** – for example, reminder of high school – You may wish to find a body positive environment to workout in. Or try group classes, yoga studio, start off at home, beginners running group.

OVERCOMING MY BARRIERS

Using the table below, have a go at troubleshooting your own barriers.

AREA OF CONCERN	HOW I WILL ADDRESS THIS

DISCOVERING JOY IN MOVEMENT

Now we will explore the many ways you can move. I'll also discuss the types of exercise that you may find trigger the dieting mentality, so that you can be on the lookout for this mentality creeping back in.

Think back to a time when you enjoyed movement. This may be all the way back in primary or elementary school and that is ok. What did you like doing at that age? Dance, gymnastics, climbing, running?

COMMON TYPES OF EXERCISE

Here are some common types of exercise you may wish to try:

- Group classes, like Les Mills are great for beginners, instructor, range of activities, online and in person. What I will say, is beware of calorie talk in some of these classes! I've reached a stage in my recovery process where I can just roll my eyes at any talk about calories, because I know better, but you may not feel like you're quite at that stage yet.
- Boxing, martial arts (contact or non-contact)
- Running, walking, hiking, rock climbing (groups or lone)
- Gardening
- Calming, slow movements yoga, Pilates, tai chi
- Dance - different types of dance (Zumba, ballet, salsa, ballroom, club, pole)
- Team sports - football, rugby, badminton, tennis
- Weightlifting - can do this in a class environment like body pump for guidance or have a PT guide you. can be done at home if you have the equipment and knowledge.
- Swimming

THINKING OUTSIDE THE BOX (OR GYM!)

If the exercises we've just mentioned seem a little boring to you, then how about some of these ideas instead:

- Ice skating, roller skating
- Paintballing, laser quest (I used to tell my PE teacher than the only time anyone will see me run is when I'm wearing a laser pack and wielding a laser gun!)
- Surfing
- Trampoline (I love this, but since having my son I've realised I need to toughen up my pelvic floor to be able to jump without weeing myself!)
- Running around with kids in a soft play area or garden
- Walking a pet
- Video games - Zumba, Just Dance, Wii/Kinect games

TRIGGERING EXERCISES

There are some exercises you may not find so pleasurable or feel triggered by. Often these focus on burning calories and can trigger the dieting mindset. They also tend to be repetitive! Some examples include:

- Cardio gym machines (no wonder people refer to the treadmill as the 'dreadmill')
- workout DVDs (yoga as an exception) certainly avoid anything by a celebrity or the type of personal who is obsessed with diets and drastic weight loss (Jillian Michaels, we are looking at you here!)
- I also strongly recommend that you avoid wearing fitness trackers, as these often encourage the calories in/calories out mindset. There are some watches on the market that will track running times and distances and lap counters for swimming, and these are fine if you're trying to improve your times for an event or just want to have a fitness goal to aim for, but please try to avoid getting one with a calorie counting function.

On the next page, I would like you to take some time to note down your preferences for exercise, such as indoor/outdoor, team sport/individual, or group/lone

You may also wish to note down your thoughts on the following:

- Can you fit the activity into your current lifestyle, or realistically make time for it how often could you do the activity?
- Can you do it at home, or do you want to attend a class, gym, or sports hall for it, if so, how close are these to you?
- Financial cost – so what is your budget?
- Can you find a way to do it for free if money is a concern?
- What is your current fitness level?
- Do you require guidance and instruction?
- And finally, what do you need to get started? clothing, shoes, equipment etc.

MY EXERCISE PREFERENCES

☐ Indoor ☐ Outdoor
☐ Team Sport ☐ Individual
☐ Group ☐ Lone

OTHER CONSIDERATIONS:

DURATION, LOCATION & FREQUENCY:

BUDGET & COST:

MY CURRENT FITNESS LEVEL & KNOWLEDGE:

WHAT I NEED TO GET STARTED:

HOW OFTEN SHOULD YOU EXERCISE?

Hopefully by now you've thought of some types of exercises you might enjoy and could happily make a regular part of your life. By this stage you may be wondering how often is ideal to be exercising. Let's look at the official guidelines.

NHS GUIDELINES FOR ADULTS AGED 19-64

To stay healthy, adults aged 19-64 should try to be active daily. This doesn't have to be a formal workout! This could be walking the dog, cleaning the house, chasing around after a toddler, or gardening.

If trying to fit something in daily stresses you out, they also suggest that you aim for at least **150 minutes of moderate aerobic activity** such as cycling or brisk walking **every week**, (this includes cycling, walking, dance, swimming etc.).

You can split these 150 minutes up however you want, say two lots of 1-hour long Zumba classes and half hour swim each week. Or to keep it very simple, aim for 30 minutes of exercise, 5 days a week.

It is also recommended that you engage in **strength exercises on two or more days a week** that work all the major muscles (legs, hips, back, abdomen, chest, shoulders, and arms).

This might look like two Les Mills Body Pump classes a week, or lifting weights in the gym, kettlebell, body weight exercises or even yoga.

Reference: https://www.nhs.uk/Livewell/fitness/Pages/physical-activity-guidelines-for-adults.aspx

DON'T TURN THESE GUIDELINES INTO RULES!

Now I do not want you to look at these guidelines, turn them into rules and panic about whether you can meet them!

Remember: any amount of activity is better than none! This is so important, because if you go all or nothing on this, you are treating exercise in the same way as food when dieting. This isn't about pass or fail.

Start off small, just one gym class a week or try 10 minutes of a yoga video on YouTube each morning, making it a part of your routine.

As you discover different forms of movement and gradually build up your fitness levels, you can start to add in more physical activity when you feel ready.

DAILY PLANNER: JOYFUL MOVEMENT

For the next 30 days, take a few minutes each day to complete these planner pages. Use the next 30 days to explore different forms of movement and what feels good for you.

Day 1	Today's Date:
Today I am feeling…	
Today I am grateful for…	
Did you move your body for the joy of it today? What kind of movement was it?	
How did you feel beforehand?	
How did you feel afterwards? What did you like or dislike about it?	

Day 2	Today's Date:
Today I am feeling…	
Today I am grateful for…	
Did you move your body for the joy of it today? What kind of movement was it?	
How did you feel beforehand?	
How did you feel afterwards? What did you like or dislike about it?	

Day 3	Today's Date:
Today I am feeling…	
Today I am grateful for…	
Did you move your body for the joy of it today? What kind of movement was it?	
How did you feel beforehand?	
How did you feel afterwards? What did you like or dislike about it?	

Day 4	Today's Date:
Today I am feeling…	
Today I am grateful for…	
Did you move your body for the joy of it today? What kind of movement was it?	
How did you feel beforehand?	
How did you feel afterwards? What did you like or dislike about it?	

Day 5	Today's Date:
Today I am feeling…	
Today I am grateful for…	
Did you move your body for the joy of it today? What kind of movement was it?	
How did you feel beforehand?	
How did you feel afterwards? What did you like or dislike about it?	

Day 6	Today's Date:
Today I am feeling…	
Today I am grateful for…	
Did you move your body for the joy of it today? What kind of movement was it?	
How did you feel beforehand?	
How did you feel afterwards? What did you like or dislike about it?	

Day 7	Today's Date:
Today I am feeling…	
Today I am grateful for…	
Did you move your body for the joy of it today? What kind of movement was it?	
How did you feel beforehand?	
How did you feel afterwards? What did you like or dislike about it?	

Day 8	Today's Date:
Today I am feeling...	
Today I am grateful for...	
Did you move your body for the joy of it today? What kind of movement was it?	
How did you feel beforehand?	
How did you feel afterwards? What did you like or dislike about it?	

Day 9	Today's Date:
Today I am feeling…	
Today I am grateful for…	
Did you move your body for the joy of it today? What kind of movement was it?	
How did you feel beforehand?	
How did you feel afterwards? What did you like or dislike about it?	

Day 10	Today's Date:
Today I am feeling…	
Today I am grateful for…	
Did you move your body for the joy of it today? What kind of movement was it?	
How did you feel beforehand?	
How did you feel afterwards? What did you like or dislike about it?	

Day 11	Today's Date:
Today I am feeling…	
Today I am grateful for…	
Did you move your body for the joy of it today? What kind of movement was it?	
How did you feel beforehand?	
How did you feel afterwards? What did you like or dislike about it?	

Day 12	Today's Date:
Today I am feeling…	
Today I am grateful for…	
Did you move your body for the joy of it today? What kind of movement was it?	
How did you feel beforehand?	
How did you feel afterwards? What did you like or dislike about it?	

Day 13	Today's Date:
Today I am feeling...	
Today I am grateful for...	
Did you move your body for the joy of it today? What kind of movement was it?	
How did you feel beforehand?	
How did you feel afterwards? What did you like or dislike about it?	

Day 14	Today's Date:
Today I am feeling…	
Today I am grateful for…	
Did you move your body for the joy of it today? What kind of movement was it?	
How did you feel beforehand?	
How did you feel afterwards? What did you like or dislike about it?	

Day 15	Today's Date:
Today I am feeling…	
Today I am grateful for…	
Did you move your body for the joy of it today? What kind of movement was it?	
How did you feel beforehand?	
How did you feel afterwards? What did you like or dislike about it?	

Day 16	Today's Date:
Today I am feeling…	
Today I am grateful for…	
Did you move your body for the joy of it today? What kind of movement was it?	
How did you feel beforehand?	
How did you feel afterwards? What did you like or dislike about it?	

Day 17	Today's Date:
Today I am feeling…	
Today I am grateful for…	
Did you move your body for the joy of it today? What kind of movement was it?	
How did you feel beforehand?	
How did you feel afterwards? What did you like or dislike about it?	

Day 18	Today's Date:
Today I am feeling…	
Today I am grateful for…	
Did you move your body for the joy of it today? What kind of movement was it?	
How did you feel beforehand?	
How did you feel afterwards? What did you like or dislike about it?	

Day 19	Today's Date:
Today I am feeling…	
Today I am grateful for…	
Did you move your body for the joy of it today? What kind of movement was it?	
How did you feel beforehand?	
How did you feel afterwards? What did you like or dislike about it?	

Day 20	Today's Date:
Today I am feeling…	
Today I am grateful for…	
Did you move your body for the joy of it today? What kind of movement was it?	
How did you feel beforehand?	
How did you feel afterwards? What did you like or dislike about it?	

Day 21	Today's Date:
Today I am feeling...	
Today I am grateful for...	
Did you move your body for the joy of it today? What kind of movement was it?	
How did you feel beforehand?	
How did you feel afterwards? What did you like or dislike about it?	

Day 22	Today's Date:
Today I am feeling…	
Today I am grateful for…	
Did you move your body for the joy of it today? What kind of movement was it?	
How did you feel beforehand?	
How did you feel afterwards? What did you like or dislike about it?	

Day 23	Today's Date:
Today I am feeling...	
Today I am grateful for...	
Did you move your body for the joy of it today? What kind of movement was it?	
How did you feel beforehand?	
How did you feel afterwards? What did you like or dislike about it?	

Day 24	Today's Date:
Today I am feeling…	
Today I am grateful for…	
Did you move your body for the joy of it today? What kind of movement was it?	
How did you feel beforehand?	
How did you feel afterwards? What did you like or dislike about it?	

Day 25	Today's Date:
Today I am feeling…	
Today I am grateful for…	
Did you move your body for the joy of it today? What kind of movement was it?	
How did you feel beforehand?	
How did you feel afterwards? What did you like or dislike about it?	

Day 26	Today's Date:
Today I am feeling...	
Today I am grateful for...	
Did you move your body for the joy of it today? What kind of movement was it?	
How did you feel beforehand?	
How did you feel afterwards? What did you like or dislike about it?	

Day 27	**Today's Date:**
Today I am feeling...	
Today I am grateful for...	
Did you move your body for the joy of it today? What kind of movement was it?	
How did you feel beforehand?	
How did you feel afterwards? What did you like or dislike about it?	

Day 28	Today's Date:
Today I am feeling…	
Today I am grateful for…	
Did you move your body for the joy of it today? What kind of movement was it?	
How did you feel beforehand?	
How did you feel afterwards? What did you like or dislike about it?	

Day 29	**Today's Date:**
Today I am feeling…	
Today I am grateful for…	
Did you move your body for the joy of it today? What kind of movement was it?	
How did you feel beforehand?	
How did you feel afterwards? What did you like or dislike about it?	

Day 30	Today's Date:
Today I am feeling…	
Today I am grateful for…	
Did you move your body for the joy of it today? What kind of movement was it?	
How did you feel beforehand?	
How did you feel afterwards? What did you like or dislike about it?	

SECTION 2: GENTLE NUTRITION

The relationship you have with food is just as important as what you eat.

WHAT IS GENTLE NUTRITION?

What do we mean by 'gentle nutrition'? Put simply, gentle nutrition is about eating foods that make you feel physically well *and* please your taste buds (don't eat a food you dislike, just because it's nutritious!)

Gentle nutrition is about recognizing the health benefits of foods and aiming to consume more of these foods, while at the same time, making sure we don't exclude foods with limited nutritional value.

In other words, adding foods in, rather than cutting down or taking food away.

It's important to only start diving into the ever-changing world of nutrition when you truly feel at peace with food and your body, otherwise you could end up falling into the trap of having food rules and labelling foods as 'good' or 'bad'.

INTUITIVE EATING REVISITED

After a while of practicing Intuitive and mindful eating, you will find that you can move past the stage of wanting to only eat all the foods you previous restricted. Eventually you become a little bored of these foods, even if you still enjoy them, but the cravings chapter and you start to want different foods.

If you've not already started practicing Intuitive Eating, and would like to know more about it, I encourage you to work through **The Peaceful Eating Planner,** available to order from Amazon.

If you are exercising (which hopefully you are by now), you may also feel a natural urge to want foods that give you more energy or help your muscles repair themselves.

This is where taking a gentle approach to nutrition comes in to play and forms part of having a 'health mindset', rather than a 'dieting mindset', which is what we'll discuss in this second section of this planner.

EATING VARIETY

When we talk about eating variety, what we mean is consuming food from all the food groups. Broadly speaking, we also mean hitting all our taste buds with a range of different flavours, consuming a full spectrum of different coloured fruits and vegetables, and even exploring food from all different cultures, as this can a great source of pleasure.

In a moment we're going to cover some basic nutritional guidelines. As we look at each different food group and the purpose of each, I'd like you think about the ways you can add a wider variety of food into your overall diet - fruits, vegetables, herbs, seasoning, lean meats, fish, dairy, whole grains (taking into account allergies etc.).

This is not about removing any foods, only about adding them in. As soon as we come at nutrition from a 'removal' perspective, we begin restricting.

Keep the pleasure you get from food at the forefront of your mind too, I don't want you to start eating food you dislike, just because it's nutritious. This is where food exploration comes into gentle nutrition, as we'll discuss further on.

NUTRITION 101: THE BASICS

When we speak of 'nutrients', what we are referring to are the different types of molecules found in food. Our energy and nutritional intake come from the following food groups:

- Carbohydrates
- Proteins
- Fats (these are the three types of macro nutrients, called 'macro' because we need large quantities of them)
- Vitamins and minerals (micronutrients)
- Fibre

Let us briefly look at the purpose of each of these groups and debunk a few myths about them too.

Trigger warning: Before I go any further, I also want to say that if you feel discussing nutrition in this manner will trigger any food anxieties you may have, or make you feel disconnected from food, then please consider working on body image and peaceful eating using my other planners in this series of four. All of them are available on Amazon.

CARBOHYDRATES

Carbs are converted by your body into energy. There are two types of carbohydrates: simple and complex, and both have their place in your diet. Carbs, particularly simple carbohydrates (which are single sugar molecules) are often avoided by dieters and traded out for higher fat diet.

The fear of carbs means many dieters restrict delicious 'play foods' (which we discuss later) and banish fresh fruit from their diets because this too is a simple carb. Doing this means they miss out on the vast array of vitamins and fibre found in food, and of course means that they are restricting food and missing out on the joy of eating delicious fresh fruit.

If you don't get enough carbohydrates in your diet, your body begins to cannibalism your body fat and, the bit that often gets skipped over by diet books, your muscle mass too! The loss of which, means you'll slow down your metabolism.

Your body does this so that it can dismantle the protein in your muscle and turn it into glucose (a process called gluco-neo-genesis, which literally means 'creation of new sugar').

This is where the diet books swoop in and tell you to eat much higher quantifies of protein into your diet to compensate for this effect, and then this is also the part where people stop thinking about food as 'food' and begin thinking about it as a mere food group or as a fuel source, rather than also a source of pleasure.

We're not going to be taking this approach, remember?

It hasn't worked in the past; it creates food anxieties and it leaves us restricting foods and then wanting to binge further down the line.

The bottom line is to make sure you consume carbs, both simple and complex.

PROTEINS

As we've just been discussing protein, let's discuss this next. Protein is often described as a 'building block' for our muscles, organs, hair, and nails. Remember: if you're not consuming adequate amounts of carbs, your body draws energy from your protein and fat stores.

Protein is certainly important, there's no doubt about that. But we don't need to be replacing all the foods in our diet with a protein source.

As a general guideline, it's recommended to include a protein source in *most* of your meals. Note that I didn't say *every* meal.

Over prioritizing the inclusion of protein often means not consuming an adequate amount of other nutrients in your diet which can leave you feeling physically drained and miserable.

FATS

Next up are fats. These too have many functions, but often get thrown under a bus by dieters who believe that eating fat will make them fat. We need an adequate amount of fat in our diets to absorb fat-soluble vitamins from our foods.

Not getting enough fats in our diet, means not being able to absorb fat soluble vitamins. It helps to keep us warm, protects our internal organs and is essential for the function of our brains. It increases our satiety too.

This doesn't mean we have to take fat consumption to the extreme (like we see in keto or low-carb diets). This can be just as dangerous for the body as not taking in enough fat.

I recommend listening to your body's cues and guidance for cravings. After recovering from food restriction and practicing intuitive eating for a while, your body will begin to guide you to the nutrition you require, so you don't need to worry about macronutrients or anything like that.

VITAMINS AND MINERALS

These are essential for bone health, hormone production, brain function, immune system and repairing cell damage. You don't need to become obsessed with getting vitamins and minerals into your overall diet. The basic nutritional guidelines, alongside your own body's cues and physical cravings will steer you in the right direction. We'll discuss these guidelines in a moment.

FIBRE

The next nutritional group to be aware of is fibre. Fibre can be found in plant-based foods, such as vegetables, fruit, legumes, nuts, and wholegrains. It's essential for our digestive system.

BASIC NUTRITIONAL GUIDELINES

So, what do we do with all this information? Take from it some basic guidelines:

- Aim to eat a wide variety of colours, flavours, and world-foods. This will help ensure you get exposure to a wide range of vitamins and minerals.

- Don't restrict foods from any food group or try to overcompensate in another (protein for example) as this risk limiting foods from the other groups.

- Aim to include around 7-10 fruits and vegetables a day, but don't make this into a strict rule. The easiest way to do this is to simply add in a variety of diced vegetables into family favourites like Bolognese and Cottage Pie. Chopped fruit mixed into Greek yogurt and then frozen to make a delicious ice cream dessert is another great one to try, and smoothies with breakfast are also an easy way to do this.

- Remember it's about adding more into your diet, not thinking about taking things out of it, as this leads to feeling deprived.

WHAT ABOUT SUPPLEMENTS?

You probably don't *need* to take supplements (protein, vitamins or otherwise). A lot of this concern comes from clever marketing from health and fitness supplement companies and stores.

If you're eating a varied diet, you're probably already getting everything you need and regularly taking in a high dose of a vitamin can be very harmful to health.

Overdosing on a vitamin is unlikely to happen from food, but it's much more likely to happen when taking vitamins and using supplements, energy drinks and vitamin enhanced protein shakes.

If you think you may be lacking in something, please consult a GP for a blood test and/or a registered dietitian.

NUTRITIOUS FOOD & PLAY FOOD

What do we mean by 'nutritious foods' and 'play foods'? And why do we need both?

Our society tends to categorize foods as either being 'healthy' or 'junk' and tends to add a moral value to eating them. I'm sure you've heard someone say, or maybe even said the words yourself, "I'm being good today and eating a salad", for example, or "I'm being naughty and having chocolate". It's often the case that the food we really love, is considered 'sinful'. A perfect example of this is 'Devil's Food Cake'!

Adding moral value to food or implying that eating less-nutritious food is pointless, makes for a very complicated relationship with food, so from this point forwards, I would like you to swap out the terms 'healthy' and 'junk' and replace them with 'nutritious' and 'play food'. In doing this, you are recognizing the nutritional benefits of nutritious foods, and recognizing the psychological benefits of eating play food, for its pleasure factor.

THE VALUE OF PLAY FOOD

Including play food in your diet is about finding a balance. It's discovering a happy medium between enjoying nutritious foods and their physical benefits, and enjoying play food, without feelings of guilt and fully engaging with the pleasurable experience of eating it. In other words, it's about seeing food for what it is: a source of both pleasure and fuel for our bodies. Food doesn't have to be one or the other, it can be both!

Once you've made peace with food, it'll no longer be the case that you'll only ever want play food. If you're listening to your body's signals, you'll also begin to want to eat other foods, and find that you crave less play food because you're no longer restricting it.

RECOMMENDATIONS FOR THIS STAGE

By this point I recommend learning some new recipes, trying new foods, and discovering new ways to enjoy a wide variety of foods - both play foods and nutritious.

I also recommend that you get your recipes and food inspiration from chefs, not diet books! These are much more likely to taste better and truly satisfy you and they don't come with a serving of body shaming either! You can also adapt your recipes over time with trial and error to add in a wider variety of ingredients, season food to taste or take out anything you dislike the taste of.

WHY CALORIES AND PORTION SIZES ARE IRRELEVANT

Let's address the issue of portion sizes and calorie counting, and the three main reasons why these are irrelevant for intuitive eaters.

Firstly, I'd to begin by highlighting that calorie guidelines and recommended portion sizes are based on averages, we're not all 'average' and we have different needs to each other because our bodies and lives are very different. Just because two people are the same gender, height, and weight, does not mean they have the same caloric needs!

The second reason is that the amount of food you require when you're hungry, will vary according to what else you've eaten that day, what you've been doing and the food you're about to eat. Among other factors (type of exercise, illness, menstrual cycle etc.)

Finally, trying to follow portion or calorie guidelines disrupts your intuition. You need to be listening to your hunger/fullness cues for guidance, not the packet, which is much easier to do now that you're no longer coming at this from a dieting mindset and instead, you're practicing eating intuitively and mindfully.

WHAT ABOUT COUNTING MACROS?

When I advocate for ditching calorie counting and measuring out food, some people will ask about counting macros instead.

I get why this seems like a better idea than counting calories from a nutritional perspective, but from a mindset perspective, it's just another way to diet.

It's another set of rules to follow at the end of the day, and can be a slippery slope to Orthorexia, where an individual becomes obsessed with the nutritional values of the food they eat.

THE PHYSICAL EFFECT OF FOOD

Over the next 30 days, we're going to be looking at how your food impacts you physically. Using the planner pages, you will be noting down what you've eaten and asking yourself:

- Did you enjoy this food?
- How did you feel immediately after eating it?
- How did you feel throughout the day?

DAILY PLANNER: UNCONDITIONAL PERMISSION TO EAT

For the next 30 days, take a few minutes each day to complete these planner pages.

Day 1	Today's Date:
Today I am feeling…	
Today I am grateful for…	
Which foods made you feel energised today? Did any make you feel sluggish?	
Which foods did you find enjoyable?	
Which foods kept you feeling full until your next meal? Did any leave you feeling empty after just a few hours?	

Day 2	Today's Date:
Today I am feeling…	
Today I am grateful for…	
Which foods made you feel energised today? Did any make you feel sluggish?	
Which foods did you find enjoyable?	
Which foods kept you feeling full until your next meal? Did any leave you feeling empty after just a few hours?	

Day 3	Today's Date:
Today I am feeling…	
Today I am grateful for…	
Which foods made you feel energised today? Did any make you feel sluggish?	
Which foods did you find enjoyable?	
Which foods kept you feeling full until your next meal? Did any leave you feeling empty after just a few hours?	

Day 4	Today's Date:
Today I am feeling...	
Today I am grateful for...	
Which foods made you feel energised today? Did any make you feel sluggish?	
Which foods did you find enjoyable?	
Which foods kept you feeling full until your next meal? Did any leave you feeling empty after just a few hours?	

Day 5	Today's Date:
Today I am feeling…	
Today I am grateful for…	
Which foods made you feel energised today? Did any make you feel sluggish?	
Which foods did you find enjoyable?	
Which foods kept you feeling full until your next meal? Did any leave you feeling empty after just a few hours?	

Day 6	Today's Date:
Today I am feeling…	
Today I am grateful for…	
Which foods made you feel energised today? Did any make you feel sluggish?	
Which foods did you find enjoyable?	
Which foods kept you feeling full until your next meal? Did any leave you feeling empty after just a few hours?	

Day 7	Today's Date:
Today I am feeling…	
Today I am grateful for…	
Which foods made you feel energised today? Did any make you feel sluggish?	
Which foods did you find enjoyable?	
Which foods kept you feeling full until your next meal? Did any leave you feeling empty after just a few hours?	

Day 8	Today's Date:
Today I am feeling…	
Today I am grateful for…	
Which foods made you feel energised today? Did any make you feel sluggish?	
Which foods did you find enjoyable?	
Which foods kept you feeling full until your next meal? Did any leave you feeling empty after just a few hours?	

Day 8	Today's Date:
Today I am feeling…	
Today I am grateful for…	
Which foods made you feel energised today? Did any make you feel sluggish?	
Which foods did you find enjoyable?	
Which foods kept you feeling full until your next meal? Did any leave you feeling empty after just a few hours?	

Day 9	Today's Date:
Today I am feeling…	
Today I am grateful for…	
Which foods made you feel energised today? Did any make you feel sluggish?	
Which foods did you find enjoyable?	
Which foods kept you feeling full until your next meal? Did any leave you feeling empty after just a few hours?	

Day 10	Today's Date:
Today I am feeling…	
Today I am grateful for…	
Which foods made you feel energised today? Did any make you feel sluggish?	
Which foods did you find enjoyable?	
Which foods kept you feeling full until your next meal? Did any leave you feeling empty after just a few hours?	

Day 11	Today's Date:
Today I am feeling…	
Today I am grateful for…	
Which foods made you feel energised today? Did any make you feel sluggish?	
Which foods did you find enjoyable?	
Which foods kept you feeling full until your next meal? Did any leave you feeling empty after just a few hours?	

Day 12	**Today's Date:**
Today I am feeling...	
Today I am grateful for...	
Which foods made you feel energised today? Did any make you feel sluggish?	
Which foods did you find enjoyable?	
Which foods kept you feeling full until your next meal? Did any leave you feeling empty after just a few hours?	

Day 13	**Today's Date:**
Today I am feeling…	
Today I am grateful for…	
Which foods made you feel energised today? Did any make you feel sluggish?	
Which foods did you find enjoyable?	
Which foods kept you feeling full until your next meal? Did any leave you feeling empty after just a few hours?	

Day 14	**Today's Date:**
Today I am feeling…	
Today I am grateful for…	
Which foods made you feel energised today? Did any make you feel sluggish?	
Which foods did you find enjoyable?	
Which foods kept you feeling full until your next meal? Did any leave you feeling empty after just a few hours?	

Day 15	**Today's Date:**
Today I am feeling…	
Today I am grateful for…	
Which foods made you feel energised today? Did any make you feel sluggish?	
Which foods did you find enjoyable?	
Which foods kept you feeling full until your next meal? Did any leave you feeling empty after just a few hours?	

Day 16	Today's Date:
Today I am feeling…	
Today I am grateful for…	
Which foods made you feel energised today? Did any make you feel sluggish?	
Which foods did you find enjoyable?	
Which foods kept you feeling full until your next meal? Did any leave you feeling empty after just a few hours?	

Day 17	Today's Date:
Today I am feeling…	
Today I am grateful for…	
Which foods made you feel energised today? Did any make you feel sluggish?	
Which foods did you find enjoyable?	
Which foods kept you feeling full until your next meal? Did any leave you feeling empty after just a few hours?	

Day 18	Today's Date:
Today I am feeling…	
Today I am grateful for…	
Which foods made you feel energised today? Did any make you feel sluggish?	
Which foods did you find enjoyable?	
Which foods kept you feeling full until your next meal? Did any leave you feeling empty after just a few hours?	

Day 19	Today's Date:
Today I am feeling…	
Today I am grateful for…	
Which foods made you feel energised today? Did any make you feel sluggish?	
Which foods did you find enjoyable?	
Which foods kept you feeling full until your next meal? Did any leave you feeling empty after just a few hours?	

Day 20	Today's Date:
Today I am feeling…	
Today I am grateful for…	
Which foods made you feel energised today? Did any make you feel sluggish?	
Which foods did you find enjoyable?	
Which foods kept you feeling full until your next meal? Did any leave you feeling empty after just a few hours?	

Day 21	**Today's Date:**
Today I am feeling…	
Today I am grateful for…	
Which foods made you feel energised today? Did any make you feel sluggish?	
Which foods did you find enjoyable?	
Which foods kept you feeling full until your next meal? Did any leave you feeling empty after just a few hours?	

Day 22	Today's Date:
Today I am feeling…	
Today I am grateful for…	
Which foods made you feel energised today? Did any make you feel sluggish?	
Which foods did you find enjoyable?	
Which foods kept you feeling full until your next meal? Did any leave you feeling empty after just a few hours?	

Day 23	Today's Date:
Today I am feeling…	
Today I am grateful for…	
Which foods made you feel energised today? Did any make you feel sluggish?	
Which foods did you find enjoyable?	
Which foods kept you feeling full until your next meal? Did any leave you feeling empty after just a few hours?	

Day 24	**Today's Date:**
Today I am feeling…	
Today I am grateful for…	
Which foods made you feel energised today? Did any make you feel sluggish?	
Which foods did you find enjoyable?	
Which foods kept you feeling full until your next meal? Did any leave you feeling empty after just a few hours?	

Day 25	**Today's Date:**
Today I am feeling...	
Today I am grateful for...	
Which foods made you feel energised today? Did any make you feel sluggish?	
Which foods did you find enjoyable?	
Which foods kept you feeling full until your next meal? Did any leave you feeling empty after just a few hours?	

Day 26	Today's Date:
Today I am feeling…	
Today I am grateful for…	
Which foods made you feel energised today? Did any make you feel sluggish?	
Which foods did you find enjoyable?	
Which foods kept you feeling full until your next meal? Did any leave you feeling empty after just a few hours?	

Day 27	**Today's Date:**
Today I am feeling…	
Today I am grateful for…	
Which foods made you feel energised today? Did any make you feel sluggish?	
Which foods did you find enjoyable?	
Which foods kept you feeling full until your next meal? Did any leave you feeling empty after just a few hours?	

Day 28	Today's Date:
Today I am feeling…	
Today I am grateful for…	
Which foods made you feel energised today? Did any make you feel sluggish?	
Which foods did you find enjoyable?	
Which foods kept you feeling full until your next meal? Did any leave you feeling empty after just a few hours?	

Day 29	Today's Date:
Today I am feeling…	
Today I am grateful for…	
Which foods made you feel energised today? Did any make you feel sluggish?	
Which foods did you find enjoyable?	
Which foods kept you feeling full until your next meal? Did any leave you feeling empty after just a few hours?	

Day 30	Today's Date:
Today I am feeling…	
Today I am grateful for…	
Which foods made you feel energised today? Did any make you feel sluggish?	
Which foods did you find enjoyable?	
Which foods kept you feeling full until your next meal? Did any leave you feeling empty after just a few hours?	

SECTION 3: ALTERNATIVE WAYS TO MEASURE HEALTH

Weight and BMI are not reliable indicators of health

ALTERNATIVE WAYS TO MEASURE HEALTH

In this part of the planner, we are going to be discussing some alternative ways to assess your health.

Typically, people use the scale, tape measures and other weight and size related metrics to assess their health. But these will only give you a small part of the overall picture of your health.

These are also the kinds of metrics people become obsessed, or anxious over and consequently begin dieting to change the metrics.

BIOMARKERS

Other metrics, or 'biomarkers', which can be easily measured at home, tell you so much more about your health.

Knowing them might even save your life, by helping you prevent or even reverse serious health conditions.

I'm not being dramatic here. In the UK for example, a shocking 1 in 74 of us have undiagnosed diabetes Type 2, according to research by diabetes.org. Diabetes Type 2 is a condition which can be easily detected with a simple prick of the finger and a blood glucose reading.

Once you know you have the condition or even if you find out that you're pre-diabetic, your GP or health care provider can help you manage the condition, and in some circumstances even reverse it entirely.

WEIGHT AS A RISK FACTOR

Please remember that when discussing the risk factors of the health conditions, it is more important to focus on lifestyle changes you can make, rather than focusing on weight loss.

Many conditions can be reversed or managed with gentle nutrition and joyful exercise. A small amount of weight loss (some studies say just 3-5% of body weight) may also be enough to significantly reduce factors – so there is certainly no need to diet or have a goal weight.

I highly recommend reading Linda Bacon's book, *Health at Every Size*, for an in depth look into the research on this.

VITAL NUMBERS

There are three vital health readings you may wish to keep a check on as these are used to directly diagnose common health conditions, sometimes even long before you know you have them.

These three readings are: blood pressure, blood glucose and blood cholesterol and we'll look at each of these in depth shortly.

If you are already aware of an issue with one or more of these readings, it's likely that your GP may have already given you a device to use at home to keep a check on it. This could be a cholesterol monitor, glucose monitor or an electronic blood pressure machine.

If you are not aware of any existing health issues, I strongly advise that you book yourself in with the GP or your local pharmacist for a health check. Explain to them that you are looking to improve your general health and be sure to inform them of any family history of diabetes, hypertension, heart problems, stroke etc.

You can buy monitors online and, in the shops, to keep a check on these numbers if you wish. I would recommend a blood pressure monitor as these are a one-off expense, whereas the blood glucose and cholesterol monitors require refills of test trips and needles which can be costly and need to be disposed of safely!

Of course, if the GP provides you with your own monitor(s) as a result of a diagnosed health issue, then any required refills are available on repeat prescription and the used needle collection service is available on the NHS.

BLOOD PRESSURE

This is the easiest reading to take from home, using a blood pressure cuff.

Your blood pressure reading consists of two numbers. The first number is larger, this is referred to as your systolic blood pressure. This is the pressure of your heart pumping blood out.

The second, smaller number is your diastolic blood pressure, which is the pressure of your heart resting.

Your blood pressure will therefore be presented to you in the format of "120/80" for example, with 120 being the systolic and 80 being the diastolic.

Blood Pressure

WHAT DOES MY READING MEAN?

A normal blood pressure reading falls within the 90/60 to 140/90. Higher than 140/90 is considered high and requires medical advice as this increases your risk of having a stroke or heart attack.

Lower than 90/60 is considered low blood pressure, which is normally ok, providing you are not experiencing symptoms such as fainting or dizziness.

If you are concerned, then please do not hesitate to see your GP for advice!

Blood pressure can change throughout the day as a reaction to stress, it can also be elevated temporarily in periods of illness.

If you have high blood pressure on a long-term basis, you may be prescribed medication for hypertension and/or advised to quit smoking, reduce salt and caffeine intake and take up more exercise which has been shown to reduce high blood pressure very effectively.

I can say from personal experience that exercise and gentle adjustments in diet can certainly make a positive difference to blood pressure on a long-term basis!

BLOOD GLUCOSE

Your blood glucose level can be used to diagnose pre-diabetes and diabetes and is also vital to keep a check on if you are managing the condition, whether Type 1 or Type 2.

If you are concerned that you may have diabetes or are at risk of it, please go to your GP as soon as possible for a formal diagnosis and medical advice. It is a serious condition and requires careful monitoring and management.

As I said earlier, there is 1 in every 74 of us walking around with diabetes, completely undiagnosed.

You are at an increased risk if you are sedentary, have a family history of diabetes, suffer with PCOS, have had gestational diabetes, or have any other existing health conditions, including those that affect the heart and kidneys.

Blood Glucose

WHAT DOES MY RESULT MEAN?

For diagnosing diabetes, blood glucose is often taken first thing in the morning, before you have eaten anything. This is referred to as a 'fasting' reading. NICE guidelines recommend that the fasting result is below 5.5 mmol/L, as any higher puts you at risk of developing Type 2.

You will be diagnosed as having pre-diabetes if your level is between 6.1 – 6.9 mmol/L and diabetes is diagnosed at 7mmol/L and above.

Anything below 4 mmol/L is low blood glucose.

Bottom line: an ideal blood glucose reading after 8 hours of fasting is a result **between 4 mmol/L and 5.5 mmol/L.**

BLOOD CHOLESTEROL

The final reading to have taken, is your blood cholesterol. High cholesterol is another serious condition, which left unchecked can lead to fatal strokes and heart attacks. To give you an example of just how serious this really is, my late father suffered with vascular dementia as a direct result of a stroke caused by a piece of cholesterol breaking off in the brain.

So, you're going to get yours tested by your GP or pharmacist, right? Great.

When you have your cholesterol level checked, you may be provided with several different readings. Usually you will be told your total cholesterol level and your LDL level. Other readings may include your HDL level and your cholesterol ratio.

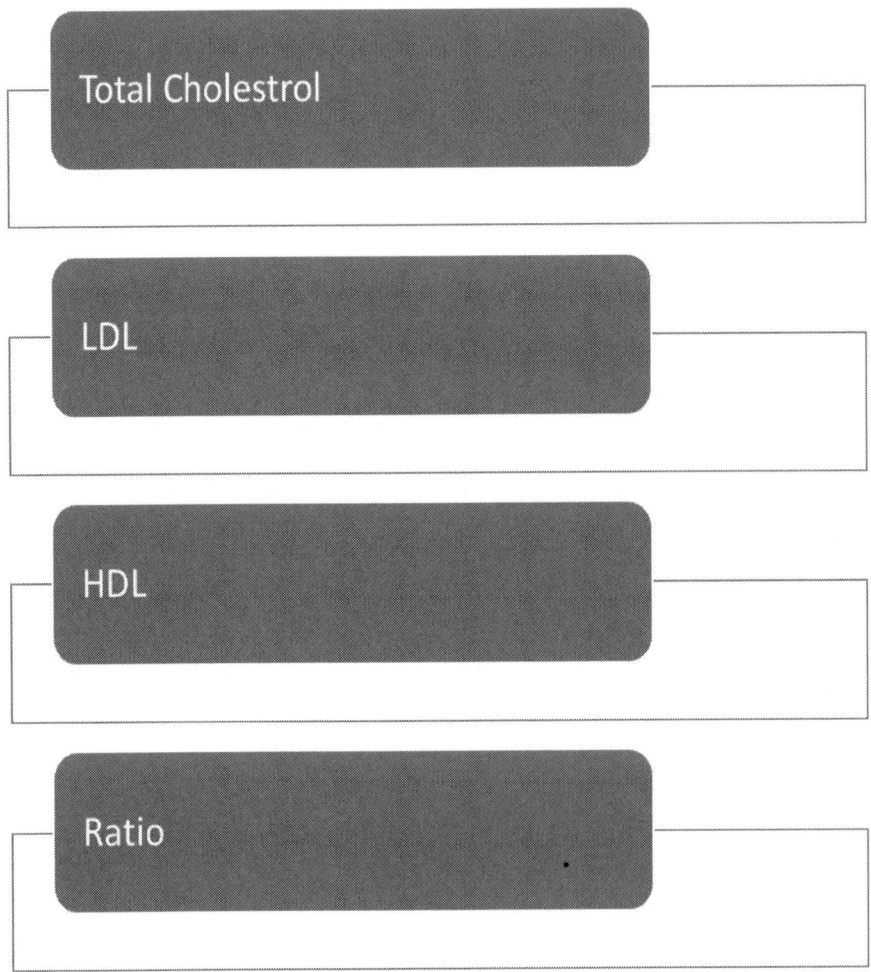

WHAT DO MY RESULTS MEAN?

Total Cholesterol: Ideally this should be **5 mmol/L or less** for healthy adults, or 4 mmol/L or less for adults considered to be of high risk (for example, those who smoke, have high blood pressure, family history of high cholesterol, stroke or heart attack).

LDL: LDL stands for Low-density lipoprotein. This is a type of protein that carries cholesterol to cells. If there is an excess of cholesterol, then it begins to build up in the arteries, causing them to narrow and increases the risk of stroke and heart attack. For this reason, it's referred to as the 'bad cholesterol'. An ideal level of LDL for a healthy adult is **3 mmol/L or less** and for those who are high-risk, 2 mmol/L or less.

HDL: HDL stands for High-density lipoprotein. This type is considered the 'good cholesterol' as its role is to carry excess cholesterol from cells back to the liver where it can be passed out of the body or broken down. An ideal level of HDL is **over 1 mmol/L**.

Cholesterol Ratio: This is your total cholesterol level, divided by your HDL level. The lower the ratio, the lower your risk of heart disease and stroke. Ideally this level will be **below 4**.

YOUR NEXT STEPS

Your next step is to book an appointment with a GP or Pharmacist for an overall heath check.

Remember: You can ask not to be weighed or stand backwards on the scale and ask to not be told your result.

If you are weighed at your appointment for any reason, please remind yourself that this number is just a piece of information, it's not an overall picture of your health and it does not define you as a person. Remember that many health conditions can be improved with changes to lifestyle.

Intuitive eating, mindfulness, gentle nutrition, joyful movement and developing effective coping strategies for emotions are all brilliant ways to improve your physical and mental health, which is what all my workbooks and online courses are based on.

OTHER WAYS TO IMPROVE HEALTH

Gentle nutrition and joyful movement will have a positive impact on your health, but please keep in mind that there are many other factors which impact your health including those out of your control, such as genetics, systemic racism, homophobia, sexism, poverty and social inequalities.

Below I've listed a few suggestions for other ways to improve your physical and mental health. Keep these in mind as you complete the next 30 days of planner pages.

- Book and regularly attend dentist and optician check-ups in addition to attending doctors' appointments when needed.

- Drink plenty of water throughout the day to stay hydrated.

- Maintain a good sleep routine (even at weekends or on days off!)

- Make time to see friends and family who are a positive influence on your mood and mindset.

- Have a list of go-to hobbies for when your mental health is in decline and you need to manage stress or anxiety.

- Have a morning routine to get you in the right mindset for the day ahead and an evening routine to wind you down for a restful night's sleep.

- Spend time outdoors and in nature.

Many of these will sound common sense, but how many of them are you making sure you're doing on a regular basis?

DAILY PLANNER: ALTERNATIVE WAYS TO LOOK AFTER HEALTH

For the next 30 days, take a few minutes each day to complete these planner pages.

Day 1	Today's Date:
Today I am feeling…	
Today I am grateful for…	
Today I cared for my physical health by…	
Today I cared for my mental health by…	
Something I can do tomorrow to look after my health in a compassionate and gentle way is…	

Day 2	Today's Date:
Today I am feeling…	
Today I am grateful for…	
Today I cared for my physical health by…	
Today I cared for my mental health by…	
Something I can do tomorrow to look after my health in a compassionate and gentle way is…	

Day 3	Today's Date:
Today I am feeling…	
Today I am grateful for…	
Today I cared for my physical health by…	
Today I cared for my mental health by…	
Something I can do tomorrow to look after my health in a compassionate and gentle way is…	

Day 4	Today's Date:
Today I am feeling…	
Today I am grateful for…	
Today I cared for my physical health by…	
Today I cared for my mental health by…	
Something I can do tomorrow to look after my health in a compassionate and gentle way is…	

Day 5	Today's Date:
Today I am feeling…	
Today I am grateful for…	
Today I cared for my physical health by…	
Today I cared for my mental health by…	
Something I can do tomorrow to look after my health in a compassionate and gentle way is…	

Day 6	Today's Date:
Today I am feeling…	
Today I am grateful for…	
Today I cared for my physical health by…	
Today I cared for my mental health by…	
Something I can do tomorrow to look after my health in a compassionate and gentle way is…	

Day 7	Today's Date:
Today I am feeling…	
Today I am grateful for…	
Today I cared for my physical health by…	
Today I cared for my mental health by…	
Something I can do tomorrow to look after my health in a compassionate and gentle way is…	

Day 8	Today's Date:
Today I am feeling…	
Today I am grateful for…	
Today I cared for my physical health by…	
Today I cared for my mental health by…	
Something I can do tomorrow to look after my health in a compassionate and gentle way is…	

Day 9	Today's Date:
Today I am feeling…	
Today I am grateful for…	
Today I cared for my physical health by…	
Today I cared for my mental health by…	
Something I can do tomorrow to look after my health in a compassionate and gentle way is…	

Day 10	Today's Date:
Today I am feeling…	
Today I am grateful for…	
Today I cared for my physical health by…	
Today I cared for my mental health by…	
Something I can do tomorrow to look after my health in a compassionate and gentle way is…	

Day 11	Today's Date:
Today I am feeling…	
Today I am grateful for…	
Today I cared for my physical health by…	
Today I cared for my mental health by…	
Something I can do tomorrow to look after my health in a compassionate and gentle way is…	

Day 12	Today's Date:
Today I am feeling…	
Today I am grateful for…	
Today I cared for my physical health by…	
Today I cared for my mental health by…	
Something I can do tomorrow to look after my health in a compassionate and gentle way is…	

Day 13	Today's Date:
Today I am feeling…	
Today I am grateful for…	
Today I cared for my physical health by…	
Today I cared for my mental health by…	
Something I can do tomorrow to look after my health in a compassionate and gentle way is…	

Day 14	Today's Date:
Today I am feeling...	
Today I am grateful for...	
Today I cared for my physical health by...	
Today I cared for my mental health by...	
Something I can do tomorrow to look after my health in a compassionate and gentle way is...	

Day 15	Today's Date:
Today I am feeling…	
Today I am grateful for…	
Today I cared for my physical health by…	
Today I cared for my mental health by…	
Something I can do tomorrow to look after my health in a compassionate and gentle way is…	

Day 16	Today's Date:
Today I am feeling…	
Today I am grateful for…	
Today I cared for my physical health by…	
Today I cared for my mental health by…	
Something I can do tomorrow to look after my health in a compassionate and gentle way is…	

Day 17	Today's Date:
Today I am feeling…	
Today I am grateful for…	
Today I cared for my physical health by…	
Today I cared for my mental health by…	
Something I can do tomorrow to look after my health in a compassionate and gentle way is…	

Day 18	Today's Date:
Today I am feeling…	
Today I am grateful for…	
Today I cared for my physical health by…	
Today I cared for my mental health by…	
Something I can do tomorrow to look after my health in a compassionate and gentle way is…	

Day 19	Today's Date:
Today I am feeling…	
Today I am grateful for…	
Today I cared for my physical health by…	
Today I cared for my mental health by…	
Something I can do tomorrow to look after my health in a compassionate and gentle way is…	

Day 20	Today's Date:
Today I am feeling…	
Today I am grateful for…	
Today I cared for my physical health by…	
Today I cared for my mental health by…	
Something I can do tomorrow to look after my health in a compassionate and gentle way is…	

Day 21	Today's Date:
Today I am feeling…	
Today I am grateful for…	
Today I cared for my physical health by…	
Today I cared for my mental health by…	
Something I can do tomorrow to look after my health in a compassionate and gentle way is…	

Day 22	Today's Date:
Today I am feeling…	
Today I am grateful for…	
Today I cared for my physical health by…	
Today I cared for my mental health by…	
Something I can do tomorrow to look after my health in a compassionate and gentle way is…	

Day 23	Today's Date:
Today I am feeling…	
Today I am grateful for…	
Today I cared for my physical health by…	
Today I cared for my mental health by…	
Something I can do tomorrow to look after my health in a compassionate and gentle way is…	

Day 24	**Today's Date:**
Today I am feeling…	
Today I am grateful for…	
Today I cared for my physical health by…	
Today I cared for my mental health by…	
Something I can do tomorrow to look after my health in a compassionate and gentle way is…	

Day 25	Today's Date:
Today I am feeling…	
Today I am grateful for…	
Today I cared for my physical health by…	
Today I cared for my mental health by…	
Something I can do tomorrow to look after my health in a compassionate and gentle way is…	

Day 26	Today's Date:
Today I am feeling…	
Today I am grateful for…	
Today I cared for my physical health by…	
Today I cared for my mental health by…	
Something I can do tomorrow to look after my health in a compassionate and gentle way is…	

Day 27	Today's Date:
Today I am feeling…	
Today I am grateful for…	
Today I cared for my physical health by…	
Today I cared for my mental health by…	
Something I can do tomorrow to look after my health in a compassionate and gentle way is…	

Day 28	Today's Date:
Today I am feeling…	
Today I am grateful for…	
Today I cared for my physical health by…	
Today I cared for my mental health by…	
Something I can do tomorrow to look after my health in a compassionate and gentle way is…	

Day 29	Today's Date:
Today I am feeling…	
Today I am grateful for…	
Today I cared for my physical health by…	
Today I cared for my mental health by…	
Something I can do tomorrow to look after my health in a compassionate and gentle way is…	

Day 30	Today's Date:
Today I am feeling…	
Today I am grateful for…	
Today I cared for my physical health by…	
Today I cared for my mental health by…	
Something I can do tomorrow to look after my health in a compassionate and gentle way is…	

END OF PLANNER REFLECTIONS

There's more to health than nutrition and fitness; your mental wellbeing, stress levels, sleep and overall life satisfaction are also important.

HEALTH BEYOND THE SCALE SELF-ASSESSMENT REVISITED

Let's see how much progress you've made over the last 90 days. Read through the statements below and tick the ones you agree with or feel apply to you most of the time.

I attend dentist, optician and doctors' appointments and check-ups whenever required.	
I am aware of my blood pressure, blood glucose, and cholesterol readings, or I get these regularly checked/monitored.	
I do not intentionally diet or weigh myself.	
Most of the time I do not allow myself to become either too hungry or too full throughout the day.	
I do not restrict particular foods or food groups (except for allergy or religious reasons).	
I take part in exercise on a regular basis which I find enjoyable.	

I make sure I get plenty of sleep at night.	
I drink plenty of water throughout the day to stay hydrated	
I have in place a network of family and friends who support me.	
I have in place a self-care routine and different hobbies which I use to manage my mental health and stress levels.	

Tally up the number of ticks and make a note of your score below. Compare this score to the score you've written down at the start of the planner to see how far you've progressed.

Today's date	
My score	

FINAL REFLECTIONS

Now that you've completed this workbook, take some time to reflect on what you've learned using the prompts below and jot your thoughts now.

- Have you found a form of movement you enjoy?

- What was your biggest barrier to exercising?

- How did you overcome this barrier?

- What are your 'play foods' and how do you feel about them these days?

- How do you feel about having a health assessment? Do you feel you can talk to your health professional without them bringing weight into the equation?

WHERE TO GO FROM HERE?

Congratulations on completing *the 90 Day Health Beyond the Scale Planner*!

Remember, your recovery doesn't end here and will be an ongoing process. Do you feel like you would benefit from more information, cognitive behavioural therapy exercises, helpful resources, and monthly support?

In *the Health Mindset Programme*™, we cover the topics of Diet Culture, Intuitive Eating, Emotional Eating and Body Positivity, in depth and in short, to-the-point, actionable video-based lessons. There's also workbooks and guides to support you in healing the relationship you have with food, exercise, and your body.

The online programme is self-paced and spaced out over 6-7 months, so you can dip in and out of it whenever you have the time. It is designed to be a safe, informative, and healing environment to enable you to recover from a lifetime of dieting and disordered eating.

It's time to make peace with food and your body and become healthy, confident, and happy.

Find out more about the 6-month online programme and join here:
https://www.beyondthebathroomscale.co.uk/thehealthmindsetprogramme/

If you haven't already, you can sign up for the free six-day taster course here: **https://www.beyondthebathroomscale.co.uk/health-mindset-starter-kit**

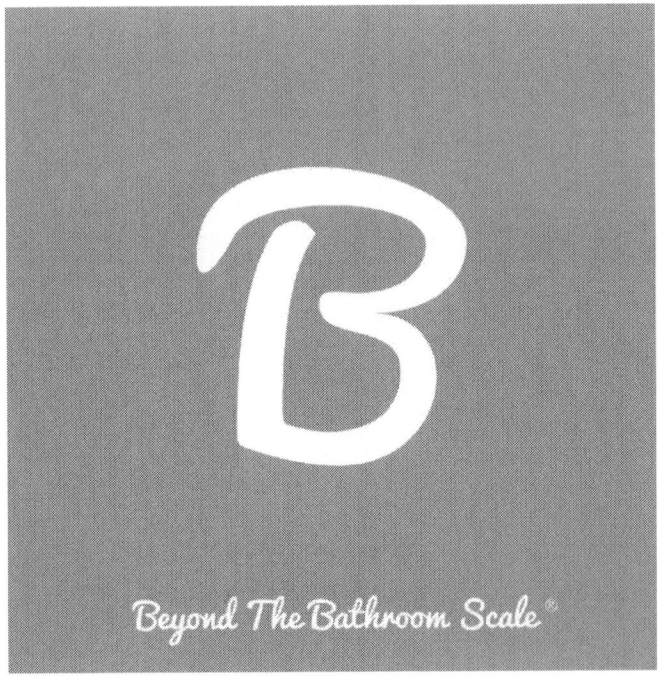

Follow on Facebook and Instagram: @Beyondthebathroomscale

Printed in Poland
by Amazon Fulfillment
Poland Sp. z o.o., Wrocław